HELPING FERTILITY IN WOMEN:
The ultimate guild on healthy fertility in women and steps to undergo.

Vanessa Smith

Table of contents

Chapter 1

Chapter 2

Chapter 3

Chapter 4

Chapter 1

Benefits of Diet,Exercise and serenity.

Exercise/physical activity during pregnancy
Being active by practicing regular moderate exercise before and after you are pregnant can help you have a healthy pregnancy and delivery. Research has shown that being active before and throughout early pregnancy may lessen your chance of developing difficulties in pregnancy, such as gestational diabetes or pre-eclampsia.

Staying strong and ready for birth
Pregnancy exerts a burden on the body. You may find it simpler to deal with if you are healthy, strong, and flexible. It has also been established that childbirth is simpler for

women who are active throughout pregnancy.

Reduced stress and anxiety

Planning to have a kid may be incredibly exciting. It may also be a tense moment for both parents-to-be. You're making arrangements for a significant shift in your life. Mental health disorders such as anxiety and sadness may be frequent in pregnancy.

Staying active may help to raise your mood and lower your chances of stress and sadness.

Health advantages for the baby

Staying active will also assist your child's long-term health. Active women are more likely to have children who are active too. It may be good for you and your spouse to consider being active as part of your planning to be parents.

Think about what type of activities you'd want to undertake when you get pregnant and when your kid comes and start doing it now. For example, it may be strolling in the park or going swimming.
You don't have to join pricey clubs or follow a specific fitness routine. It's about concentrating on methods to make movement part of daily life.

How much exercise should I be doing?
If you have always been fairly active
For most women, if you have always been active, continuing to exercise at the same level before (and throughout) pregnancy is safe and healthful.

If you workout intensely on most days of the week
A tiny percentage of women who exercise intensively on most days of the week, such as competitive athletes, may be recommended to limit their activity to a

moderate level if they are experiencing issues becoming pregnant.

If you have not been active previously, start to build up your level of activity immediately. The advice is to build up to:

at least 150 minutes of moderate aerobic activity a week and strength workouts on two or more days a week that train all the main muscles\sor:

75 minutes of intense movement a week and strength workouts on two or more days a week that train all the main muscles\sor:

a combination of moderate and strenuous aerobic activity a week and strength workouts on two or more days a week that work all the main muscles
Moderate activity implies any exercise that will elevate your heart rate, make you breathe quicker, and feel warmer. You

should still be able to converse without stopping for a breath.

Vigorous activity implies any exercise that makes you breathe hard and rapidly. If you're working at this level, you won't be able to utter more than a few words without halting for air.

Good examples include

Race
Walking,
Jogging
Running
Tennis.
Dancing
Gardening.

Avoid sitting down as much as possible
Cut decrease the amount of time you spend sitting down (being sedentary).

You might also try:

1: walking or cycling to work\standing on the bus or train, or getting off a stop earlier early/going to a co-worker's desk instead of emailing or calling\setting a reminder on your phone to get up regularly\staking the stairs instead of the elevator or escalator.

2: Try an app, such as Couch to 5k or Active 10

These NHS applications allow thousands of individuals who never imagined they could be active to start on the path to fitness.

3: Head to the park on your lunch break

If there is one near you. If not, take a stroll. Don't spend your luncheon sitting down at your desk if feasible.

4: If you have additional children, walk them to school, preschool, or toddler group if it's not too far

Turning something that occurs every day into physical activity is a wonderful method to become more active. And it will keep your youngsters fit too.

5: Get a step-counting app for your phone

By tracking your steps and delivering modest prizes they show you how much you are accomplishing and aid with motivation.

Chapter 2

Understanding fuss and fertility.

It is vital to understand what happened to the body during adolescence and a woman's menstrual cycle, how a woman's reproductive system operates, and how general health and welfare are related to fertility and the reproductive system.

Understanding the anatomy and the biology of reproduction can impact choices about avoiding pregnancy and choosing whether and when to get pregnant. The next portions examine the foundations of puberty, the menstrual cycle, what it means to have fertility awareness, and apply fertility awareness-based approaches (FABM) to family planning, and infertility in women and men.

Puberty:

Puberty is the time in life when a kid reaches sexual maturity. This suggests that the hormone levels in the body—estrogen, and progesterone in females and testosterone in boys—increase and cause physical and emotional changes to occur. Puberty generally occurs between years 8 and 13 for females and ages 10 and 15 for boys, and the process affects boys and girls differently. When girls hit puberty, they generally start their menstrual cycle.

Menstrual Cycle

The menstrual cycle refers to the monthly process that happens in a woman's body to prepare for a future pregnancy. It includes the release of an egg from the ovaries (called ovulation), changes in the cervix and thickening of the uterine wall, several hormonal changes, and shedding of the thicker uterine wall by bleeding (called menstruation, sometimes known as a "period" or "menses"). Hormonal fluctuations produce the alterations that occur during the menstrual cycle. If pregnancy does not occur, the body removes the extra lining of the uterus. The blood and tissue leave the uterus through the cervix and exit the body via the vagina. The length of the menstrual cycle is the number of days commencing from the first day when bleeding starts until the first day of the following month when bleeding begins again.

Finest practice and mistakes.

Regular menstrual periods occurring in the years between adolescence and menopause are often an indicator that the female body is working normally. Some women have challenges with menstruation, such as irregular or heavy, painful periods; this may be an indication of a health condition. Many women also endure premenstrual syndrome (PMS) symptoms. Women having period issues or PMS should talk to a healthcare practitioner about techniques to manage these symptoms.

In addition to the hormonal changes and the changes happening inside the body, females may also feel alterations in their vaginal discharge. Vaginal discharge is fluid—usually white or clear—that pours out of the vagina. Most females have vaginal discharge. The amount and consistency of vaginal discharge vary at different points in a female's cycle. Increased vaginal discharge may be caused by normal menstrual cycle changes, vaginal infection, or cancer (rare) (rare) (rare).

Unusual vaginal discharge may also be an indication of pelvic inflammatory disease (PID), a sickness of a female's reproductive systems often caused by numerous sexually transmitted infections (STIs) (STIs) (STIs). If a female has more than her regular amount of vaginal discharge, she may need to visit her healthcare expert.

How to Chart Menstrual Cycles

To track her menstrual cycle, a woman may simply write the day her period starts and when it stops on a paper or electronic calendar. Smartphone and PC tools that monitor menstrual periods are also available. Over time, this monitoring will assist a woman to understand what the usual amount of time between periods is, which may help her estimate when her next period will start.

Tracking the menstrual cycle could yield vital information for conversations with healthcare practitioners. For example, a patient may desire to discuss the length of her period or her experiences with pain or profuse bleeding during her cycle. In addition, tracking the cycle is vital to anticipating ovulation, which may inform decisions about when to have intercourse, and whether the intention is to avoid pregnancy or become pregnant.

Fertility Awareness

Fertility awareness is being aware of the menstrual cycle and the changes in a woman's body that happens during this time and knowing when a woman is most likely to get pregnant. Women and couples become better familiar with the indications of ovulation and the regularity of the menstrual cycle to understand how to plan a sexual activity to avoid pregnancy or get pregnant.

Fertility Awareness-Based Methods (FABM) of Family Planning

Fertility awareness-based techniques (FABM) require a woman to learn to recognize the signals of her fertile days, which are the days of each month in which she is most likely to become pregnant (conceive) (conceive) (conceive). Based on her aims, she may want to have unprotected sex during this period to conceive, or she may attempt to avoid pregnancy by not having intercourse or by employing a barrier birth control device, such as condoms, during this time.

There are several fertility awareness-based techniques that women may apply, such as the following:

Natural family planning
Standard days or calendar method
Cervical mucous method
Basal body temperature method
Ovulation technique
Symptothermal technique (combining the previous approaches) (combining the other methods) (combining the other methods)
Infertility
Infertility is characterized as not being able to become pregnant despite having regular intercourse (sex) without birth control after one year (or after six months if a woman is 35 or older) (or after six months if a woman is 35 or older) (or after six months if a woman is 35 or older). Infertility is frequent. Out of 100 couples in the United States,

around 12 to 13 of them have issues becoming pregnant.

About one-third of infertility cases are caused by reproductive issues in women and another one-third of infertility cases are attributed to fertility problems in males. The remaining occurrences are caused by a mix of male and female illnesses or by issues that cannot be verified.

Infertility in Women

Most incidences of female infertility are caused by difficulties with ovulation. Ovulation difficulties may be caused by hormone imbalances from a variety of sources. Although less common, clogged fallopian tubes may also cause female infertility. If the fallopian tube is clogged owing to sickness, surgery, or other obstacles, then sperm cannot reach the egg to fertilize it.

Other less prevalent explanations of reproductive troubles in women can include physical abnormalities with the uterus or uterine fibroids, which are non-cancerous tumors composed of fibrous tissue and muscle cells that grow on the walls of the uterus

Chapter 3

Best exercise to apply.

Moderate kinds of exercise for five hours or less per week are normally suggested for healthy women of all body types while you're TTC. If you generally go hard and heavy in your exercise activities, consider stepping down on intensity. Replace your rigorous activity with one of these suggested workouts:

WALKING: is always a safe approach to doing your workout. It's wonderful for your cardiovascular system, improves endurance, is low-impact, and is a terrific stress-buster.
DANCING: helps you bust a move and boost blood flow. Dancing also gives a considerable calorie burn.

BICYCLING: 30 minutes a couple of times a week is an excellent method to get your exercise done. Just make sure you're safe;

wear a helmet and look out for irresponsible drivers if you're sharing the road. apply Yoga may be a terrific technique to limber yourself (excellent for delivering a baby!) and relax.

A yoga body is powerful and elegant, and yoga may surely help you cope with the stress of infertility. Whether you practice yoga at home or work out in a studio, don't push your body too far. Also, Bikram (hot yoga) may not be suggested. Consult your doctor.
Pilates is another good strategy to keep fit and boost your fertility. Pilates is soothing, yet delivers a challenge.

SWIMMING: fitness is one of the finest methods to work out while you're TTC. You can get a solid aerobic exercise without placing too much stress on your joints. Swimming for fitness enables you to pick the most comfortable speed and build on it.

This is a good alternative for individuals just beginning an exercise regimen.

Always listen to your body, and keep hydrated. You never want to put yourself in danger for a fall, or injury, and remember you might get pregnant at any moment, so go easy if you aren't into regular exercise.

RUNNERS

For those who run marathons frequently, you may need to table your training for just a little. Intense, long-distance running might interfere with ovulation from time to time therefore it's advisable to postpone any marathon preparation for the time being. When you've been striving to get pregnant, to no effect, you may feel as if your body is beyond your control. Moderate exercise, in this scenario, may be extremely powerful in easing the stress of infertility. When you combine frequent (more than 1 hour per week, less than 5) exercises with a nutritious diet you're taking charge of your body and giving your future kid a healthy, happy parent.

Chapter 4

Finest practice and mistakes.

1. Not Knowing When You Ovulate

If you can recall back to 5th-grade sex ed, many women have a 28-day cycle, which means for them, ovulation normally occurs on day 14. But don't think that time clock necessarily applies to you. Individual cycles vary, so you may have one that's somewhat shorter or longer. To find out the precise day you ovulated, you'd need to count 14 days back from the day you began your period. (That's because although not everyone ovulates on the 14th day of your cycle, your period nearly always arrives 14 days following ovulation.) Use our Ovulation Predictor tool to help you forecast when you'll ovulate next.

2. Having Sex Only on the Day of Ovulation

When it comes to trying to conceive, timing is everything–but that doesn't mean you have only one chance at creating a kid! When you ovulate, the discharged egg may survive in the fallopian tube for 12 to 24 hours. There, it may meet up with any accessible sperm, which can normally survive in a woman's body for about three days and occasionally as long as five. That implies your viable window is possibly six days—the four days coming up to ovulation, the day you ovulate, and the following day. Of those, you're most fertile between the two to three days before ovulation and the day of ovulation itself.

3. Having Sex Every Day

Believe it or not, too much sex may lower your man's sperm count, which can then take a few days to recoup. Doctors suggest

Once you have your ovulation time down, having sex every
other day, instead of every day, during your reproductive window.

4. Obsessing About Positions

If you've resorted to standing on your head, raising your legs in the air, or bending into any other coital or post-coital posture to improve your baby-making prospects, we've got some news for you: You may be wasting your time. (Nope, you don't need to be a contortionist to become pregnant after all.) The reality is, that the bulk of a man's sperm moves toward the woman's egg the instant he ejaculates. As about the left-over liquid that comes out after? It won't truly have much sperm left in it anyhow. So if you want to do it missionary-style or position a cushion under your hips, go right ahead—but don't worry yourself out over it too much. Your prospects of becoming pregnant rely on many more elements than simply sheer posture.

5. Hanging onto Unhealthy Habits
It's a no-brainer that you'd have to abandon those unhealthy behaviors like smoking, drinking, and drug usage if you got pregnant. But remember those lifestyle variables might impact your fertility too.

In addition to giving up smoking, drug use, and heavy drinking, aim to eat a healthy diet, exercise in moderation, try to get your weight into a healthy range, and ease up on caffeine.

If you're under 35, it's not unusual for it to take up to a year to become pregnant, It's also totally natural to feel disappointed after a few months—but if you don't have any underlying health concerns, you should wait it out before seeking the advice of a fertility doctor. 80 percent of healthy patients will become pregnant during this period. If you're over 35, go ahead and set up an appointment with a specialist after you've been trying for six months, instead of a year. We realize, that sometimes the wait might drive you insane

7. Waiting Too Long to See a Specialist,

there are undoubtedly exceptions to the one-year-wait rule: If your cycle is shorter than 25 days or longer than 35 days, if you experience painful or heavy periods, or if you've had a serious pelvic infection in the past, it's a good idea to get to the doctor sooner rather than later to get things checked out. One more crucial reason to not put off a doctor's appointment? If you have a history of STDs. Even if you only believe you've been exposed to one, it's better to get checked out ASAP.

8. Assuming the 'Problem' Is with You

A lot of couples concentrate their fertility inquiry on the woman, but Felix points out that 40 percent of the time, reproductive difficulties might be related to the guy. So if you haven't conceived after a year of trying and are under 35, you should both go to the doctor. Your spouse will require a semen study to rule out any difficulties on his end

9. Waiting Too Long to Try
We get it—you probably have a lot left on that pre-baby to-do list (establishing a career, beefing up your savings, buying a bigger house, etc). (establishing a career, beefing up your savings, buying a bigger house, etc.). But age is a factor in fertility. When you hit 35, you officially enter what's known as "advanced maternal age," a designation that recognizes the dangers of having problems conceiving–and carrying–a healthy pregnancy when you're older. According to Felix , a woman's ability to conceive decreases by about 50 percent between the ages of 20 and 40. If you're in a

stable relationship and want a child, don't wait just because you think it won't be a problem to get pregnant later in life. If you feel ready, by all means, go for it.

www.ingramcontent.com/pod-product-compliance
Lightning Source LLC
LaVergne TN
LVHW052114160826
845678LV00015B/3543

* 9 7 9 8 8 4 8 3 4 6 1 1 4 *